Stay Strong with Chair Yoga for Seniors Over 60:

The Ultimate Guide to Feeling Younger, Stronger, and Healthier with Just 10 Minutes a Day – Home Exercises for Weight Loss and Muscle Toning

BY
Elijah Finn

CONTENTS

INTRODUCTION

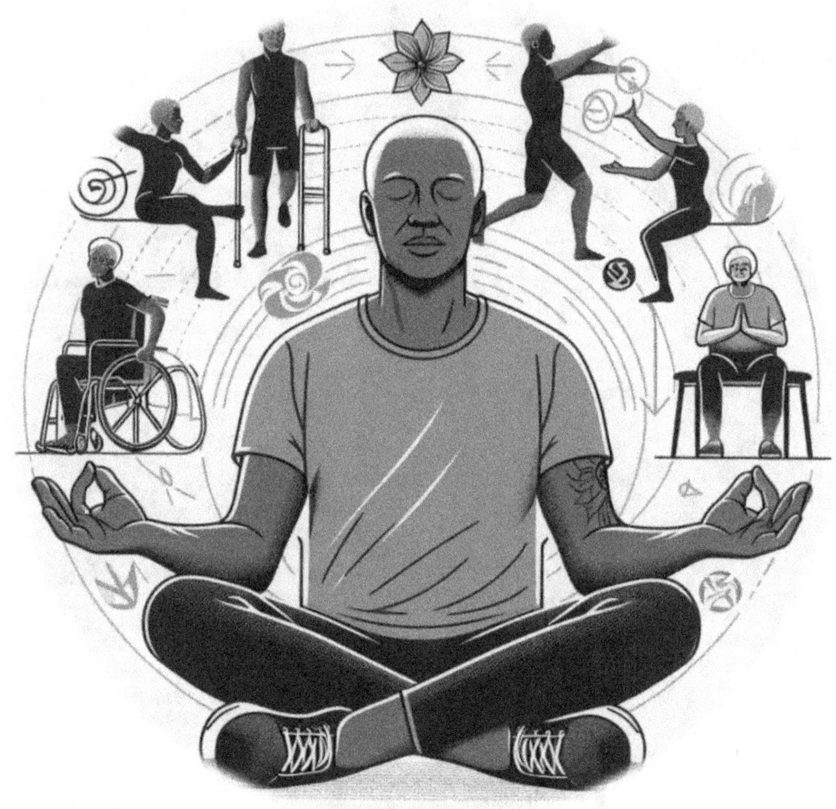

Welcome to Chair Yoga

As we age, staying active becomes increasingly important, yet many seniors face physical limitations that can make traditional exercise routines challenging. Chair yoga provides a perfect solution. Whether you're just starting your fitness journey or looking for a way to maintain your current level of activity, chair yoga is designed to be gentle on your body while offering numerous physical and mental benefits.

In this guide, we'll explore how just 10 minutes a day of chair yoga can help you feel younger, stronger, and healthier. You don't need fancy equipment or expensive gym memberships—just a chair and a small space to get started. Chair yoga is all about adapting traditional yoga postures to be performed while seated or with the support of a chair. It's especially useful for seniors because it's low-impact, safe, and effective in targeting areas like flexibility, balance, strength, and even mental well-being.

Many people are unaware of how much exercise they can actually achieve in a seated position. Chair yoga enables seniors to stay strong, improve flexibility, and enhance mobility without straining joints or risking injury. You might be surprised at how quickly you can begin to notice the benefits, even with a short daily practice. Whether you're aiming to tone your muscles, lose weight, or simply stay mobile, chair yoga can be tailored to fit your unique needs.

By the end of this guide, you'll have all the tools and knowledge to incorporate chair yoga into your daily routine, helping you feel stronger, more flexible, and more connected to your body and mind.

What is Chair Yoga?

Chair yoga is a form of yoga that adapts traditional yoga postures and movements so they can be performed while seated or with the support of a chair. This practice is incredibly accessible, making it ideal for seniors or anyone with mobility issues. Unlike standard yoga, chair yoga removes the need to get up and down from the floor, making it gentler on the joints and easier to modify based on your ability level.

Chair yoga still provides all the same benefits of traditional yoga. You can stretch, strengthen muscles, and even practice mindful breathing while seated. Because it's performed sitting down or using the chair for balance, you reduce the risk of falling or overextending muscles, which is particularly important for seniors.

Chair yoga incorporates many familiar yoga poses like seated forward bends, modified twists, and gentle backbends. You might also do standing poses like warrior or tree pose with the chair for support. This style of yoga focuses not only on stretching but also on building strength, improving balance, and helping seniors become more mindful of their movements.

Another great feature of chair yoga is that you can practice almost anywhere—at home, in a park, or even in your office—since all you need is a sturdy chair. Chair yoga isn't just physical exercise; it's also about creating a sense of mental calm and promoting emotional well-being.

What You Can Expect:
- **Gentle Stretches:** Lengthen and release tight muscles.
- **Strength Building:** Tone key muscle groups, especially those needed for stability.
- **Balance Improvement:** Reduce the risk of falls with balance exercises.

- **Stress Relief:** Incorporate deep breathing techniques and mindfulness.

Chair yoga gives you the best of both worlds: the physical benefits of yoga with the added comfort and safety of using a chair. It's a great way to stay active regardless of your age or physical condition.

Benefits of Chair Yoga for Seniors

Chair yoga offers seniors a wide range of physical and mental benefits. Whether you're looking to build strength, improve your mental clarity, or simply add a new activity to your routine, chair yoga can deliver.

➤ Physical Benefits

1. **Improved Flexibility:** Aging often leads to stiffness in the muscles and joints, but chair yoga helps seniors to gradually improve their flexibility. Gentle stretches performed in a seated position can lengthen the muscles and help keep the joints mobile, preventing them from becoming too tight.

2. **Enhanced Balance:** Chair yoga strengthens the muscles that support balance, like the core, legs, and hips. Regular practice can improve your balance and stability, reducing your risk of falls.

3. **Increased Strength:** Chair yoga isn't just about stretching — it also helps to build muscle strength, particularly in key areas like the arms, legs, and core. This can improve your ability to perform everyday tasks, from standing up out of a chair to carrying groceries.

4. Better Posture: Sitting for long periods can lead to poor posture, but chair yoga encourages you to sit up tall and engage your muscles, which helps to align your spine and improve overall posture.

5. Reduced Pain: Many seniors suffer from joint pain or arthritis, but chair yoga can help to alleviate some of this discomfort. Gentle movements increase circulation and help to lubricate the joints, easing stiffness and reducing pain over time.

6. Weight Loss: Chair yoga can be a surprisingly effective way to burn calories and help with weight management. Consistent practice helps to tone muscles, increase metabolism, and promote overall fat loss, even if you're seated.

➢ **Mental Benefits**

1. Stress Relief: Chair yoga incorporates mindful breathing and relaxation techniques that can reduce stress levels. Learning how to breathe deeply and slowly helps to activate the body's relaxation response, which calms the mind.

2. Improved Mental Clarity: Many yoga poses increase blood flow to the brain, improving cognitive function and mental clarity. Chair yoga can help you stay focused, think more clearly, and even boost memory.

3. Better Sleep: Seniors often experience disruptions in sleep as they age, but practicing chair yoga can help promote better sleep patterns. The calming nature of yoga helps prepare the body for rest, making it easier to fall and stay asleep.

4. Mood Boosting: Yoga naturally releases endorphins, the body's "feel-good" chemicals. These can boost your mood, help reduce symptoms of depression, and promote a more positive outlook on life.

Research Support and Testimonials

Research on chair yoga has shown a positive impact on seniors. A study published in the Journal of Geriatric Physical Therapy found that chair yoga improved physical function, balance, and overall quality of life in older adults. Testimonials from seniors who have incorporated chair yoga into their routine often emphasize how it helped them feel more energetic, less stiff, and more confident in their ability to move without fear of falling.

➢ **Real-Life Testimonials:**
- "I've been doing chair yoga for six months, and I'm amazed at how much stronger I feel. I used to struggle with standing for long periods, but now I can move around with ease."
- "Chair yoga has become a lifesaver for me! It's helped me reduce the stiffness in my legs and improve my overall flexibility."

Getting Started

Before you dive into chair yoga, it's essential to set yourself up for success by preparing your environment and body.

➢ ## Choosing a Chair

Your chair will be your most important tool, so choose one that's sturdy and comfortable. Here are some things to consider:

- Chair Height: Ideally, your chair should allow your feet to be flat on the floor, with your knees bent at a 90-degree angle. If your feet don't reach the floor, use a yoga block or a thick book for support.
- Back Support: The chair should have a supportive backrest, but it should not be too soft or cushioned. You need a firm chair to help you maintain proper posture.
- No Wheels: Avoid using a chair with wheels, as this can make the chair unstable during movements. A kitchen or dining chair works best.

Finding a Quiet Space

Set up your chair in a location where you won't be disturbed. Make sure you have enough space around you to move freely, especially if you'll be incorporating standing poses or movements that require reaching out. A quiet environment will also help you focus on your breath and relaxation.

Preparing Your Body

Warm up your body before beginning your practice by doing a few gentle stretches or walking around the room for a few minutes. Focus on relaxing any tense areas, like your shoulders or neck. Pay attention to how your body feels and listen to any signs of stiffness or discomfort. Chair yoga should feel gentle and enjoyable.

Safety Considerations

Although chair yoga is designed to be a safe and low-impact form of exercise, it's still essential to follow some basic safety guidelines to avoid injury.

Listen to Your Body

Your body will tell you what it can handle, so it's crucial to pay attention to how you feel during each movement. If you experience pain, stop immediately and either rest or modify the pose to make it more comfortable. Don't push yourself to the point of discomfort.

Avoid Overstretching

It's easy to get carried away when you're feeling good, but be mindful not to overstretch. The goal is to gently stretch the muscles, not to force them into positions they aren't ready for. Start small and build up gradually as you become more flexible.

Use Modifications

Don't hesitate to modify the poses to fit your needs. For example, if a particular movement feels difficult, use props like cushions or folded towels for extra support. Chair yoga is all about adapting the poses to work for you.

Consult Your Doctor

Before beginning any new exercise program, especially if you have existing health conditions, it's always a good idea to check in with your doctor. They can help you determine whether chair yoga is appropriate for you and offer advice on modifications based on your specific needs.

Move Slowly and Mindfully

Perform each pose slowly and with intention. Quick, jerky movements can lead to injury, while slow, controlled movements allow you to stay in tune with your body and prevent strain.

In conclusion, chair yoga is a versatile, accessible, and incredibly beneficial form of exercise for seniors. Whether you're looking to improve your physical health or boost your mental well-being, chair yoga offers an easy and effective way to stay strong and feel younger with just a few minutes a day. So grab a chair, find a peaceful spot, and start your journey toward better health today!

Part 1: Warming Up

Chapter 01

Neck and Shoulder Stretches

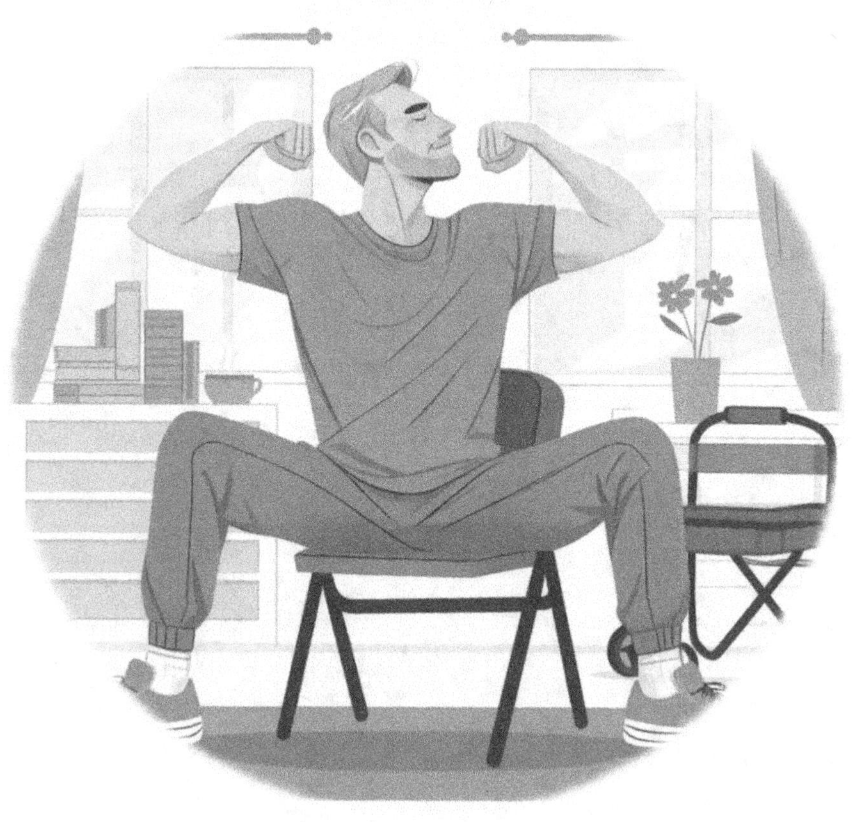

A significant portion of tension tends to accumulate in the neck and shoulders, particularly as we age. The repetitive movements or, conversely, long periods of inactivity we experience can lead to stiffness and pain in these areas. In this chapter, we'll focus on gentle neck and shoulder stretches that are essential for releasing this tension and increasing flexibility. By incorporating these stretches into your chair yoga routine, you'll notice improvements in posture, range of motion, and overall relaxation.

The exercises outlined in this chapter will take just a few minutes but can have a profound impact on how you feel throughout the day. The stretches are designed to be accessible and easy to follow, even for those with limited mobility.

Neck Circles

➢ **Why It's Important:**
The neck area often holds a lot of tension, especially due to long periods of looking down at phones, computers, or even books. Over time, this can lead to stiffness, headaches, and limited range of motion. Neck circles are a gentle, circular movement that helps to warm up the muscles of the neck and increase flexibility, making it easier to move your head without discomfort.

➢ **How to Perform Neck Circles:**
1. Sit upright in your chair with your feet flat on the floor and your spine straight.
2. Relax your shoulders, letting them fall away from your ears.

3. Close your eyes or keep them softly focused straight ahead.
4. Begin by gently dropping your chin toward your chest, feeling a gentle stretch in the back of your neck.
5. Slowly, start to rotate your head to the right side, bringing your ear toward your right shoulder (don't force your head too far down—just go as far as feels comfortable).
6. Continue the circle, tilting your head backward, and then bring your left ear toward your left shoulder.
7. Finally, bring your head forward, returning to the starting position with your chin toward your chest.
8. Repeat the circular motion 3–5 times in this direction, then switch directions, performing 3–5 circles in the opposite direction.

➤ Tips for Neck Circles:

- Move slowly and with intention. Quick movements can lead to strain or dizziness.
- Keep the movement gentle and within your comfortable range of motion. If you experience any pain, stop and reduce the range of motion.
- Focus on deep, slow breaths as you perform the circles. This will help your body relax and release tension more effectively.

➤ Benefits:

- Increased neck flexibility and mobility.
- Relief from tension headaches and stiff necks.
- Promotes better posture, reducing the forward head position many people develop over time.

Shoulder Shrugs

➢ Why It's Important:

Shoulder shrugs are a simple yet powerful movement that helps to release tension in the shoulders and improve circulation in the upper body. Many seniors experience shoulder tightness due to poor posture or stress. Shoulder shrugs are an easy way to relieve that tightness and reduce discomfort.

➢ How to Perform Shoulder Shrugs:

1. Sit upright in your chair with your feet flat on the floor, spine tall, and hands resting on your thighs or hanging by your sides.
2. Inhale deeply and slowly raise your shoulders toward your ears, as though you are trying to shrug.
3. Hold this position for a moment, feeling the stretch in your neck and shoulders.
4. Exhale slowly and release your shoulders downward, allowing them to fall away from your ears.
5. Repeat this motion for 8–10 repetitions, focusing on relaxing your shoulders completely each time you release them.

➢ Tips for Shoulder Shrugs:

- As you shrug your shoulders up, focus on tension release—imagine you're lifting the weight of the world off your shoulders.
- Move with the rhythm of your breath: inhale as you lift, exhale as you release.

- If your shoulders are particularly tight, try doing a gentle massage on your shoulders after each shrug for extra relaxation.

> **Benefits:**

- Helps to reduce stress and tension in the shoulders.
- Improves circulation to the upper body, aiding in flexibility and movement.
- Increases awareness of posture, which can help prevent long-term shoulder and neck problems.

Head Tilts

> **Why It's Important:**

Head tilts help to stretch the muscles along the sides and back of the neck, improving range of motion and reducing stiffness. These are particularly beneficial for individuals who spend a lot of time sitting or looking down, which can cause tightness in the neck and shoulders. Head tilts also encourage better alignment of the spine, reducing strain in the upper body.

> **How to Perform Head Tilts:**

1. Sit upright in your chair, feet flat on the floor, spine straight, and hands resting on your thighs or by your sides.
2. Inhale deeply, and as you exhale, gently tilt your head to the right, bringing your right ear toward your right shoulder. Don't force the stretch—just go as far as is comfortable.
3. Hold this position for 3–5 breaths, feeling the stretch along the left side of your neck.

4. Inhale to bring your head back to center, then repeat the tilt on the left side, bringing your left ear toward your left shoulder.
5. After completing the side-to-side tilts, you can also gently tilt your head forward, bringing your chin toward your chest to stretch the back of your neck, and then tilt your head backward to stretch the front of your neck.
6. Repeat the tilts 3–5 times on each side, moving slowly and with control.

➢ Tips for Head Tilts:

- Avoid forcing your head too far down or to the side. The movement should be gentle and controlled.
- Use deep breaths to enhance the stretch. Each time you exhale, see if you can relax your neck a little more.
- If you feel any sharp pain or discomfort, reduce the range of motion and move more slowly.

➢ Benefits:

- Increases neck mobility, allowing for greater range of motion.
- Relieves tension and stiffness, particularly from prolonged sitting or poor posture.
- Promotes better alignment of the spine, which can reduce headaches and upper back pain.

Arm Circles

➢ Why It's Important:

Arm circles are an excellent way to warm up the muscles in your shoulders, arms, and upper back. They help to increase circulation, enhance flexibility, and improve range of motion in the shoulders. Many seniors experience reduced shoulder mobility, but arm circles provide a gentle and effective way to keep these muscles flexible and strong.

> ## How to Perform Arm Circles:

1. Sit upright in your chair with your feet flat on the floor, back straight, and shoulders relaxed.
2. Extend your arms straight out to the sides at shoulder height, so that your body forms a "T" shape.
3. Begin making small, controlled circles with your arms, moving them in a forward direction. Start with circles that are about the size of a dinner plate.
4. Gradually increase the size of the circles if it feels comfortable, making larger rotations. Do this for 10–15 seconds.
5. Reverse the direction of the circles, moving your arms backward for another 10–15 seconds.
6. Lower your arms and relax for a moment before repeating the movement.

> ## Tips for Arm Circles:

- Keep your shoulders relaxed and away from your ears throughout the movement. The focus should be on the circular motion of your arms, not tension in your neck.
- Start with smaller circles and work your way up to larger ones as your shoulders warm up.
- Breathe deeply throughout the exercise, inhaling as you lift and exhaling as you lower.

> ## Benefits:

- Helps to increase shoulder mobility and prevent stiffness.
- Improves blood circulation to the upper body, which can reduce the risk of shoulder pain and injury.
- Strengthens and tones the muscles in the shoulders, helping with posture and daily activities like reaching and lifting.

Conclusion

Incorporating these simple neck and shoulder stretches into your daily routine can greatly reduce tension, improve flexibility, and increase strength in areas that are prone to stiffness. Whether you're starting your day with these movements or using them as a mid-day stretch break, you'll feel the benefits almost immediately.

By focusing on gentle, controlled movements, you can safely improve your range of motion and relieve discomfort. Remember to move slowly, listen to your body, and enjoy the process. These stretches will not only help you physically but also provide a moment of mental clarity and relaxation throughout your day.

Chapter 02

Wrist and Hand Stretches

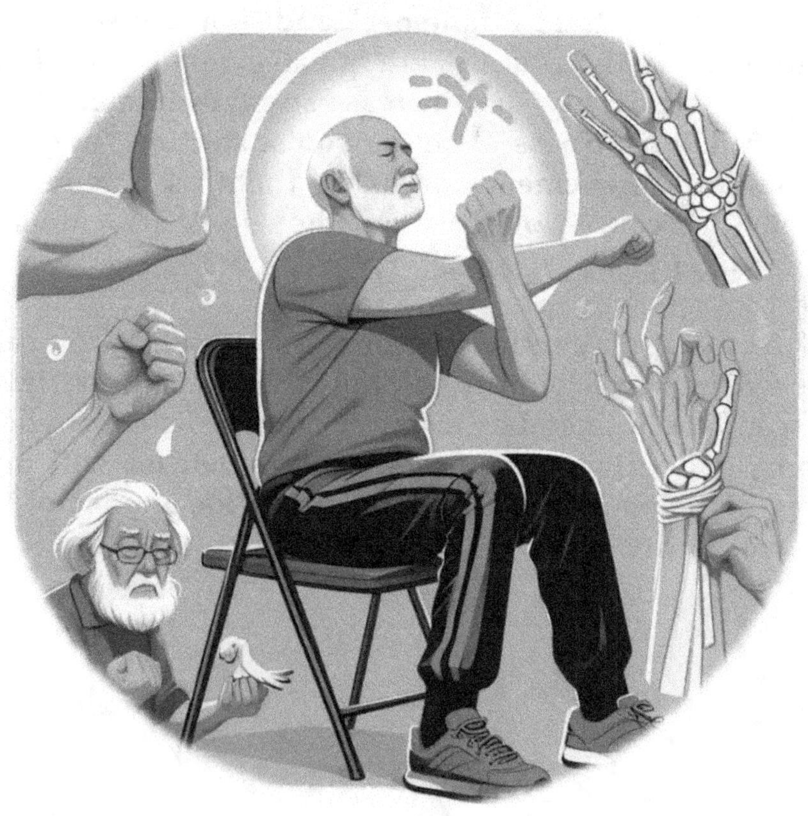

As we age, our hands and wrists can become stiff, weak, and prone to discomfort. This can be particularly concerning for seniors, who often rely on their hands for everyday activities like cooking, writing, and even using their smartphones. Fortunately, wrist and hand stretches are simple, effective exercises that can significantly enhance flexibility, dexterity, and strength in these areas. In this chapter, we'll cover three key exercises: wrist flexions and extensions, finger stretches, and hand grips. Each exercise is designed to be performed while seated in a chair, making them easy to incorporate into your daily routine.

By dedicating just a few minutes each day to these stretches, you can help maintain and improve the health of your wrists and hands, ensuring they remain functional and pain-free.

Wrist Flexions and Extensions

➤ Why It's Important:

Wrist flexions and extensions are fundamental movements that promote flexibility and strength in the wrist joint. As we use our hands throughout the day, repetitive motions can lead to stiffness or discomfort. By regularly performing these stretches, you can prevent stiffness, increase blood flow, and maintain a healthy range of motion in your wrists.

➤ How to Perform Wrist Flexions and Extensions:

1. Sit upright in your chair with your feet flat on the floor. Rest your forearms on your thighs or on the armrests, with your hands hanging over the edge.
2. Start with wrist flexion: Inhale deeply, then slowly bend your wrists so that your palms move toward your forearms. Hold this position for a moment.
3. Exhale as you gently return your wrists to the neutral position.
4. Now, move into wrist extension: Inhale and slowly extend your wrists so that your fingers point toward the floor. Hold for a moment.
5. Exhale as you return to the neutral position.
6. Repeat this process for 5–10 repetitions, focusing on the fluid motion of flexion and extension.

➢ **Tips for Wrist Flexions and Extensions:**
- Keep your movements slow and controlled to avoid strain.
- If you experience discomfort, reduce the range of motion and listen to your body.
- For added resistance, you can use a light wrist weight or squeeze a soft ball during these stretches to enhance strength training.

➢ **Benefits:**
- Increases wrist flexibility and range of motion.
- Reduces the risk of stiffness and discomfort, especially in those who engage in repetitive tasks.
- Promotes blood circulation to the wrists, helping to keep the joints healthy.

Finger Stretches

➢ **Why It's Important:**

The fingers are intricate structures that play a crucial role in our daily lives. Over time, the tendons and muscles in the fingers can become tight, leading to reduced dexterity and even pain. Finger stretches can enhance mobility, improve circulation, and help alleviate tension in the hands.

➢ How to Perform Finger Stretches:

1. Sit comfortably in your chair with your feet flat on the floor and your arms resting on your thighs.
2. Start with your right hand: Extend your fingers straight out in front of you, keeping them close together.
3. Inhale deeply and then slowly spread your fingers apart, as wide as you can without forcing them. Hold for a moment.
4. Exhale and bring your fingers back together.
5. Next, make a fist with your right hand: Inhale as you curl your fingers in toward your palm, squeezing gently.
6. Exhale as you slowly open your hand, extending your fingers fully.
7. Repeat these movements for your right hand 5–10 times, then switch to your left hand and repeat.

➢ Tips for Finger Stretches:

- Move slowly and deliberately, paying attention to how your fingers feel during each stretch.
- If you find it difficult to spread your fingers apart, use a rubber band around your fingers to provide some resistance as you stretch.
- Always listen to your body; if you feel pain or discomfort, ease up on the stretch.

➢ Benefits:

- Enhances dexterity and fine motor skills.
- Reduces tension in the hands, which can prevent conditions like carpal tunnel syndrome.
- Improves circulation and strengthens the finger muscles, making daily tasks easier and more comfortable.

Hand Grips

➤ Why It's Important:

Grip strength is a critical aspect of overall hand health, impacting everything from holding a pen to carrying groceries. As we age, our grip strength can diminish, leading to challenges in performing daily activities. Hand grip exercises are essential for strengthening the muscles in the hands and fingers, improving overall functionality.

➤ How to Perform Hand Grips:

1. Sit comfortably in your chair with your feet flat on the floor.
2. For this exercise, you can use a squeeze ball, a rolled-up towel, or even just your fist.
3. Hold the squeeze ball in your right hand and inhale as you squeeze it tightly, feeling the muscles in your hand and forearm engage.
4. Hold the squeeze for about 3–5 seconds while maintaining a steady breath.
5. Exhale as you slowly release the grip on the ball.
6. Repeat this squeezing motion for your right hand 10–15 times.
7. Switch to your left hand and perform the same squeezing action.

➢ Tips for Hand Grips:

- If you're using a towel, you can also try to twist it as you squeeze, which will engage different muscles in your hands.
- To increase the intensity of the exercise, you can use a higher resistance squeeze ball or hold the squeeze for a longer period.
- Make sure to alternate hands to ensure balanced strength development.

➢ Benefits:

- Strengthens the muscles in your hands and fingers, improving grip strength.
- Enhances overall functional ability, making it easier to perform daily tasks.
- Prevents muscle atrophy and increases endurance in hand movements.

Conclusion

Incorporating wrist and hand stretches into your daily routine is essential for maintaining mobility, strength, and flexibility in these vital areas. The exercises outlined in this chapter—wrist flexions and extensions, finger stretches, and hand grips—are not only easy to perform but also require minimal time and space, making them perfect for seniors.

By practicing these stretches regularly, you can alleviate tension, prevent stiffness, and significantly improve your grip strength. This can have a positive impact on your daily life, allowing you to engage in activities that require fine motor skills with greater ease and comfort. Remember, consistency is key; even just a few minutes each day can make a world of difference in your hand and wrist health.

Part 2:
Seated Poses

Chapter 03

Spine Twists

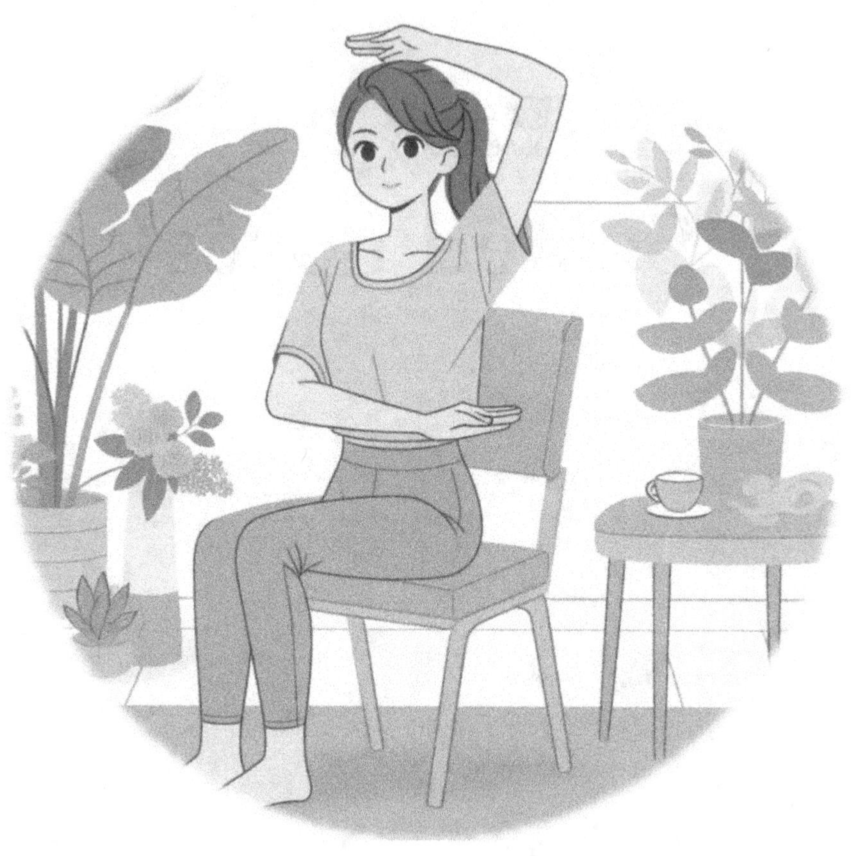

Maintaining a healthy spine is vital for overall well-being, especially as we age. The spine supports our body structure, protects our spinal cord, and allows us to perform various movements with ease. Spine twists are an excellent way to enhance spinal flexibility, improve posture, and alleviate tension in the back. In this chapter, we will focus on two essential exercises: the seated spinal twist and wrist and ankle circles. These exercises can be performed while seated in a chair, making them accessible and safe for seniors.

By integrating these stretches into your daily routine, you can promote spinal health and mobility while also preparing your wrists and ankles for movement.

Seated Spinal Twist

➢ Why It's Important:

The seated spinal twist is a powerful exercise that promotes spinal flexibility and helps relieve tension in the lower back. Twists engage the muscles of the spine, improve circulation, and can even assist in digestion by stimulating the abdominal organs. This gentle twist is ideal for seniors, as it is low-impact and can be adjusted according to individual comfort levels.

➢ How to Perform the Seated Spinal Twist:

1. Sit comfortably in your chair with your feet flat on the floor, hip-width apart. Sit tall, ensuring your back is straight and your shoulders are relaxed.
2. Inhale deeply, allowing your spine to lengthen as you lift your chest slightly.
3. Exhale and gently turn your torso to the right. Place your left hand on your right knee and your right

hand on the back of the chair or the armrest for support.

4. Hold the twist for 5–10 deep breaths, allowing your body to relax into the stretch. Focus on deepening the twist with each exhale.

5. Inhale as you return to the center, maintaining your tall posture.

6. Repeat the twist on the left side: Exhale as you turn your torso to the left, placing your right hand on your left knee and your left hand on the back of the chair.

7. Hold the twist for another 5–10 deep breaths, breathing deeply and allowing your body to ease into the position.

8. Return to the center on an inhale and relax.

> **Tips for Seated Spinal Twist:**

- If you feel any discomfort in your lower back, reduce the depth of your twist or modify the position of your hands.
- Keep your movements gentle; this is not a race. Allow your body to warm up and ease into the stretch.
- To enhance the stretch, you can focus on breathing deeply, visualizing each breath as a way to help you gently deepen the twist.

> **Benefits:**

- Increases spinal flexibility, allowing for greater ease of movement.
- Helps alleviate tension and stiffness in the back and shoulders.
- Promotes relaxation and enhances circulation to the spine and surrounding muscles.

Wrist and Ankle Circles

➤ **Why It's Important:**

Wrist and ankle circles are essential exercises that warm up the joints, improve mobility, and enhance coordination. These movements are particularly beneficial for seniors, as they help maintain joint health and prevent stiffness. Incorporating wrist and ankle circles into your routine ensures that you're not only addressing your spine but also taking care of your peripheral joints.

➤ **How to Perform Wrist and Ankle Circles:**

Wrist Circles:

1. Sit comfortably in your chair with your feet flat on the floor.
2. Extend your right arm in front of you at shoulder height, keeping your palm facing down.
3. Inhale deeply, and then slowly rotate your wrist in a circular motion clockwise for about 10 repetitions.
4. Exhale as you reverse the direction and perform 10 more rotations counterclockwise.
5. Lower your right arm and repeat the same process with your left arm.

Ankle Circles:

1. Keeping your feet flat on the floor, lift your right foot slightly off the ground.
2. Inhale and begin to rotate your ankle clockwise in a circular motion for 10 repetitions.
3. Exhale as you reverse the direction, performing 10 rotations counterclockwise.

4. Lower your right foot back to the floor and repeat the ankle circles with your left foot.

➢ Tips for Wrist and Ankle Circles:

- Keep your movements smooth and controlled to avoid strain on the joints.
- If you have any discomfort in your wrists or ankles, consider reducing the size of the circles or taking a break.
- Pay attention to your breathing; it helps promote relaxation during the exercise.

➢ Benefits:

- Improves flexibility and range of motion in the wrists and ankles, which is essential for daily activities.
- Enhances coordination and balance, reducing the risk of falls.
- Promotes circulation and warmth in the joints, preventing stiffness.

Conclusion

Incorporating spine twists into your daily routine is an effective way to maintain spinal flexibility and improve your overall posture. The seated spinal twist and wrist and ankle circles are simple exercises that require minimal time and space, making them perfect for seniors.

By dedicating just a few minutes each day to these movements, you can alleviate tension, enhance flexibility, and promote joint health. Remember that consistency is key; the more you practice these exercises, the greater the benefits you will experience. With a healthy spine and well-functioning joints, you can enjoy a more active and fulfilling lifestyle.

Chapter 04

Leg and Hip Stretches

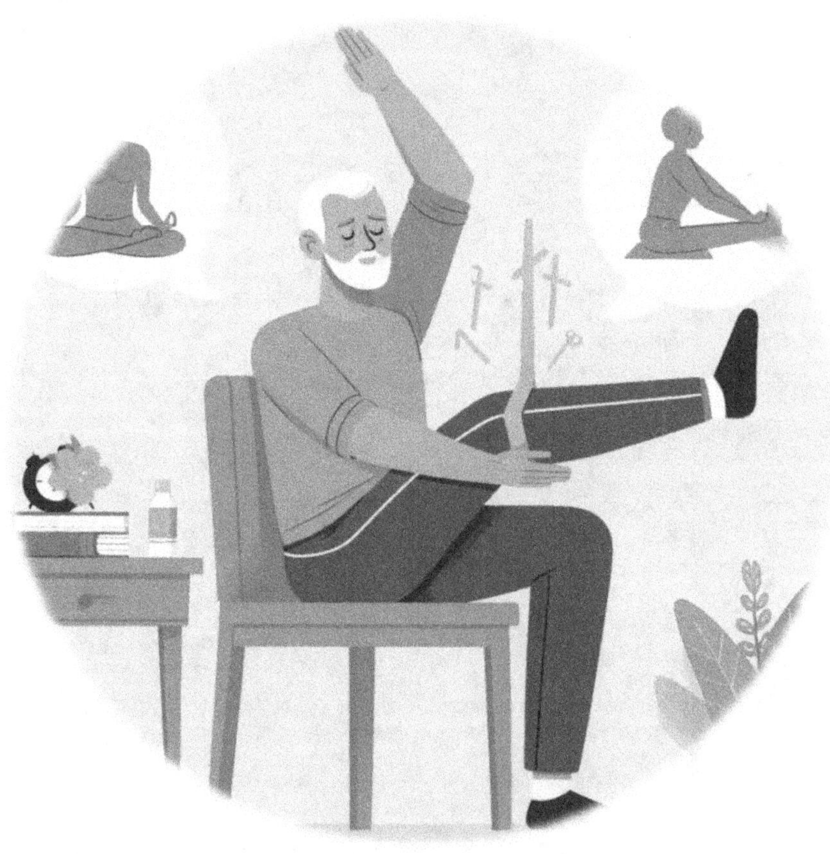

As we age, maintaining the strength and flexibility of our legs and hips becomes increasingly important. Leg and hip stretches are crucial for improving mobility, preventing falls, and enhancing overall quality of life. In this chapter, we will focus on four effective stretches: seated leg raises, hip flexor stretch, inner thigh stretch, and hamstring stretch. Each of these exercises is designed to be performed while seated in a chair, making them accessible and easy for seniors.

By regularly incorporating these stretches into your routine, you can improve circulation, strengthen your legs, and enhance your flexibility, allowing you to stay active and engaged in your daily activities.

Seated Leg Raises

➢ **Why It's Important:**
Seated leg raises are an excellent way to strengthen the muscles in your legs while improving circulation. These exercises target the quadriceps and hamstrings, enhancing your overall leg strength and stability. They are particularly beneficial for seniors, as they can help prevent muscle atrophy and maintain mobility.

➢ **How to Perform Seated Leg Raises:**
1. Sit comfortably in your chair with your back straight and your feet flat on the floor.
2. Inhale deeply and lift your right leg straight out in front of you until it is parallel to the floor. Keep your knee straight and your toes pointed.
3. Hold the position for 3–5 seconds, engaging your thigh muscles.
4. Exhale as you slowly lower your leg back to the starting position.

5. Repeat the leg raise on the right side for a total of 10–15 repetitions.
6. Switch to your left leg and repeat the process.

> ➤ **Tips for Seated Leg Raises:**
- Keep your movements slow and controlled; avoid swinging your leg.
- Engage your core muscles to maintain balance and support your back.
- If lifting your leg straight out is too challenging, you can perform the exercise with a slight bend in your knee.

> ➤ **Benefits:**
- Strengthens the leg muscles, improving mobility and stability.
- Enhances blood circulation to the legs, reducing the risk of swelling and discomfort.
- Promotes better posture and balance.

Hip Flexor Stretch

> ➤ **Why It's Important:**

The hip flexors are a group of muscles that allow you to lift your knees and bend at the waist. As we age, these muscles can become tight, leading to discomfort and limited mobility. A seated hip flexor stretch helps improve flexibility in this area, alleviating tension and enhancing overall mobility.

> ➤ **How to Perform the Hip Flexor Stretch:**

1. Sit at the edge of your chair, ensuring your back is straight and your feet are flat on the floor.
2. Inhale deeply and extend your right leg back behind you, keeping it straight and resting the top of your foot on the floor or chair.
3. Exhale as you lean slightly forward, feeling a gentle stretch in the front of your right hip. Keep your left knee over your left ankle.
4. Hold the stretch for 15–30 seconds, breathing deeply and relaxing into the position.
5. Inhale as you return to the starting position.
6. Switch to the left side and repeat the stretch.

➤ Tips for the Hip Flexor Stretch:

- Keep your movements gentle; do not force your body into the stretch.
- Focus on maintaining a straight back throughout the stretch; avoid rounding your shoulders.
- If you feel any discomfort in your knee, adjust your position to ensure your knee is properly aligned.

➤ Benefits:

- Increases flexibility in the hip flexors, allowing for greater ease of movement.
- Helps alleviate tension in the lower back, promoting better posture.
- Improves overall mobility and function, making daily activities easier to perform.

Inner Thigh Stretch

> ## Why It's Important:

The inner thighs play a crucial role in stabilizing the body and maintaining balance. As we age, flexibility in this area can diminish, leading to discomfort and increased risk of falls. A seated inner thigh stretch is an excellent way to increase flexibility and promote relaxation in the groin area.

> ## How to Perform the Inner Thigh Stretch:

1. Sit comfortably in your chair with your back straight and your feet flat on the floor.
2. Inhale deeply and slowly spread your legs apart, allowing your knees to move outward. Keep your feet firmly planted on the floor.
3. Exhale and lean slightly forward, keeping your back straight. You should feel a gentle stretch in your inner thighs.
4. Hold the stretch for 15–30 seconds, breathing deeply and relaxing into the position.
5. Inhale as you return to the starting position.

> ## Tips for the Inner Thigh Stretch:

- Only stretch as far as is comfortable; you should feel a stretch but not pain.
- If you have tightness, consider using a prop, like a cushion, to support your body as you lean forward.
- Focus on maintaining a neutral spine; avoid rounding your back.

> ## Benefits:

- Increases flexibility in the inner thighs, improving mobility.
- Enhances balance and stability, reducing the risk of falls.

- Promotes relaxation and reduces tension in the groin area.

Hamstring Stretch

➤ **Why It's Important:**

Tight hamstrings can lead to discomfort and affect your overall mobility. A seated hamstring stretch helps lengthen these muscles, improving flexibility and reducing the risk of injury. This stretch is particularly important for seniors, as maintaining hamstring flexibility can enhance daily activities such as walking and climbing stairs.

➤ **How to Perform the Hamstring Stretch:**

1. Sit at the edge of your chair with your back straight and your feet flat on the floor.
2. Extend your right leg straight out in front of you, keeping your heel on the floor and your toes pointed toward the ceiling.
3. Inhale deeply and lengthen your spine, reaching your arms forward.
4. Exhale as you lean forward gently from your hips, reaching toward your right toes. Keep your back straight; avoid rounding your shoulders.
5. Hold the stretch for 15–30 seconds, breathing deeply and relaxing into the position.
6. Inhale as you return to the starting position and switch to the left leg.

➤ **Tips for the Hamstring Stretch:**

- Only stretch as far as you can without discomfort; avoid pushing yourself too hard.
- If you cannot reach your toes, use a stretch strap or towel around your foot to assist.
- Maintain a slow and steady breath throughout the stretch.

> **Benefits:**

- Lengthens the hamstrings, improving overall leg mobility.
- Reduces the risk of injury and discomfort, especially when engaging in physical activities.
- Enhances balance and stability, contributing to improved quality of life.

Conclusion

Incorporating leg and hip stretches into your daily routine is essential for maintaining mobility, strength, and flexibility in these vital areas. The seated leg raises, hip flexor stretch, inner thigh stretch, and hamstring stretch are simple yet effective exercises that require minimal time and space.

By dedicating just a few minutes each day to these movements, you can improve circulation, enhance flexibility, and strengthen your legs and hips. Remember, consistency is key; the more you practice these stretches, the greater the benefits you will experience. With strong and flexible legs and hips, you can enjoy a more active and fulfilling lifestyle.

Part 3:
Balancing Poses

Chapter 05

Balance Exercises

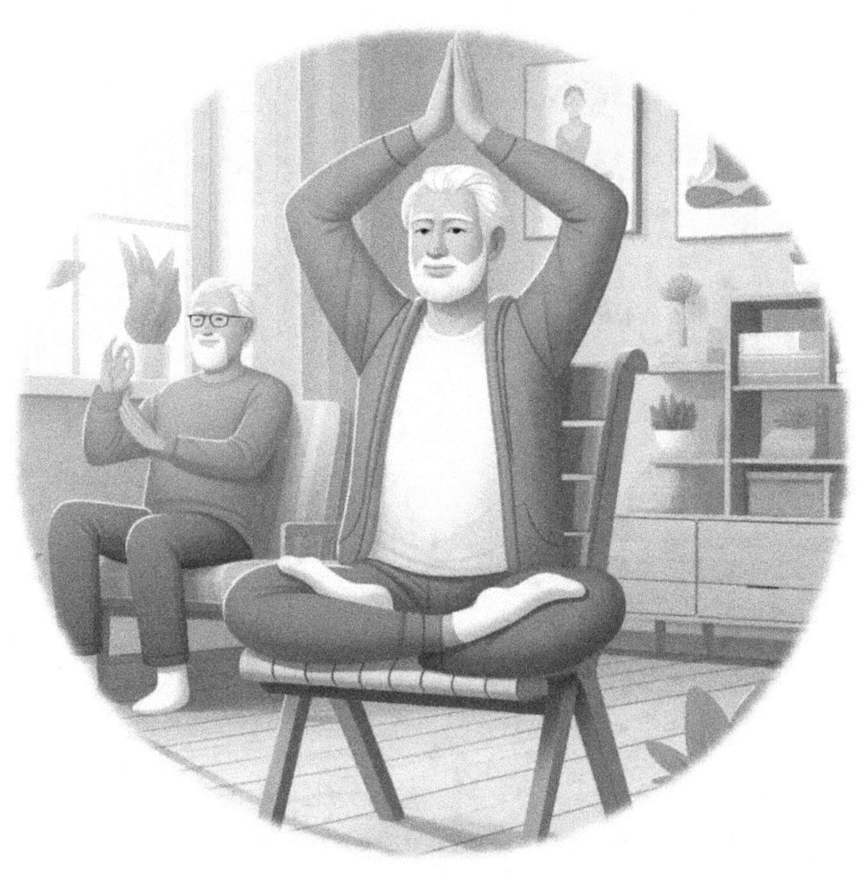

Balance is a critical component of physical health, especially as we age. Maintaining good balance can help prevent falls, enhance mobility, and improve overall quality of life. In this chapter, we will focus on three effective balance exercises: the tree pose (chair variation), single leg raises, and heel-to-toe walks. These exercises can be performed while seated or standing, making them accessible for seniors.

By incorporating these balance exercises into your routine, you can enhance your stability, strengthen your legs, and promote confidence in your movements.

Tree Pose (Chair Variation)

➤ Why It's Important:

The tree pose is a traditional yoga pose that enhances balance and stability. The chair variation allows seniors to perform this pose safely while providing support. This exercise strengthens the legs and core while promoting focus and mindfulness.

➤ How to Perform the Tree Pose (Chair Variation):

1. Sit comfortably in your chair with your feet flat on the floor and your back straight. Ensure your chair is sturdy and won't slide.
2. Inhale deeply and lift your right foot off the ground, placing the sole of your foot against your left ankle or calf. Avoid placing your foot directly on your knee to prevent pressure on the joint.
3. Once you feel stable, place your hands on your hips or bring them together in front of your chest in a prayer position.

4. Hold the position for 5–10 breaths, focusing on a point in front of you to maintain your balance.
5. Exhale as you slowly lower your right foot back to the floor.
6. Repeat the pose on the left side.

➤ Tips for the Tree Pose (Chair Variation):
- If you find it challenging to balance, use the chair back for support or place your hands on the armrests.
- Focus on engaging your core muscles to provide stability.
- Visualize your body as a tree, with your roots (feet) grounded and your branches (arms) reaching toward the sky.

➤ Benefits:
- Improves balance and stability, reducing the risk of falls.
- Strengthens the legs, core, and back muscles.
- Enhances focus and mindfulness, promoting mental well-being.

Single Leg Raises

➤ Why It's Important:
Single leg raises are a fantastic exercise for improving balance and strengthening the legs. This exercise targets the quadriceps, hamstrings, and core, enhancing stability and coordination.

➤ How to Perform Single Leg Raises:
1. Sit comfortably in your chair with your back straight and your feet flat on the floor.

2. Inhale deeply and lift your right leg straight out in front of you until it is parallel to the floor. Keep your knee straight and your toes pointed.
3. Hold the position for 3–5 seconds, focusing on maintaining your balance.
4. Exhale as you lower your leg back to the starting position.
5. Repeat the leg raise on the right side for a total of 10 repetitions.
6. Switch to your left leg and repeat the process.

➤ Tips for Single Leg Raises:

- To increase the challenge, you can hold onto the sides of the chair or keep your hands on your hips.
- Focus on engaging your core muscles to maintain stability.
- If you find it difficult to lift your leg straight out, try performing the exercise with a slight bend in your knee.

➤ Benefits:

- Strengthens the leg muscles, enhancing overall stability and balance.
- Improves coordination and body awareness.
- Promotes better posture and core strength.

Heel-to-Toe Walks

➤ Why It's Important:

Heel-to-toe walks are an excellent exercise for challenging balance and coordination. This simple movement mimics the act of walking while promoting focus and stability. Practicing this exercise can enhance your confidence in walking and daily activities.

➤ **How to Perform Heel-to-Toe Walks:**
1. Stand up from your chair, ensuring you have a sturdy support nearby if needed.
2. Inhale deeply and step forward with your right foot, placing your heel directly in front of your left toes.
3. Shift your weight onto your right foot, then bring your left foot forward, placing your heel in front of your right toes.
4. Continue this pattern, taking 5–10 steps forward.
5. To return to your starting position, turn around and repeat the exercise, stepping backward in the same heel-to-toe manner.

➤ **Tips for Heel-to-Toe Walks:**
- If you feel unsteady, perform this exercise near a wall or countertop for support.
- Focus on keeping your eyes straight ahead to improve balance and coordination.
- Take slow, deliberate steps; if you need to, pause for a moment between steps to regain your balance.

➤ **Benefits:**
- Challenges balance and coordination, reducing the risk of falls.
- Improves gait and walking stability.
- Enhances confidence in movement and mobility.

Conclusion

Incorporating balance exercises into your daily routine is essential for maintaining stability, strength, and confidence in your movements. The tree pose (chair variation), single leg raises, and heel-to-toe walks are simple yet effective exercises that can be performed with minimal space and equipment.

By dedicating just a few minutes each day to these movements, you can significantly improve your balance and coordination. Remember that consistency is key; the more you practice these exercises, the greater the benefits you will experience. With enhanced balance, you can enjoy a more active, independent, and fulfilling lifestyle.

Part 4:
Strength Training

Chapter 06

Upper Body Strength

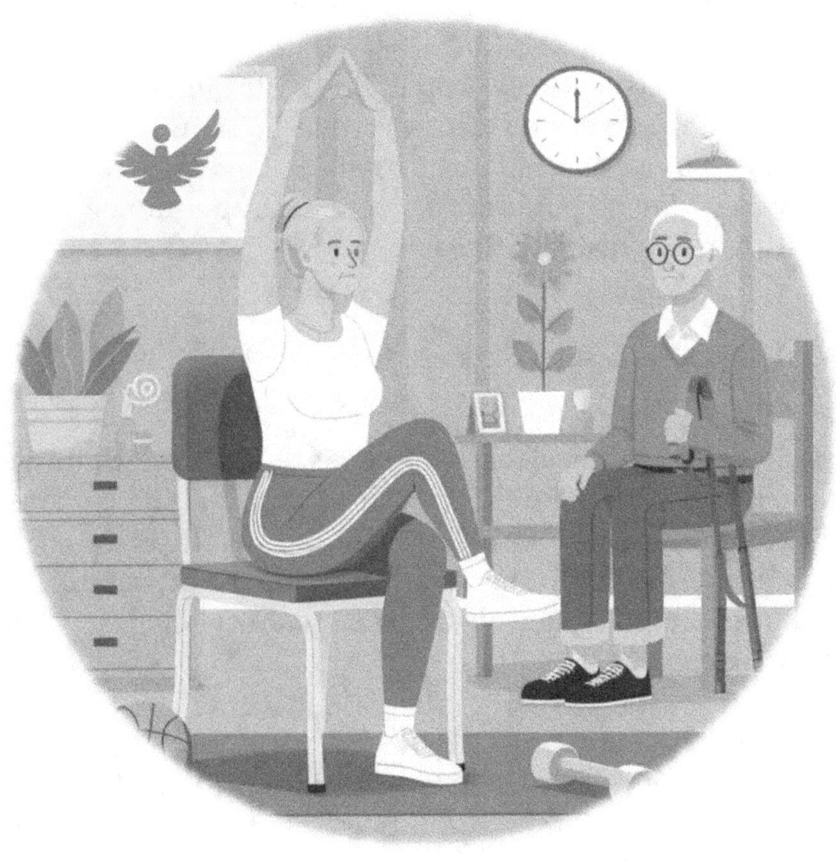

Strengthening the upper body is crucial for maintaining independence and functionality as we age. A strong upper body supports daily activities such as lifting, reaching, and even sitting up straight. In this chapter, we will explore three effective exercises for enhancing upper body strength: chair dips, seated rows, and bicep curls. Each of these exercises can be performed using minimal equipment, making them accessible and manageable for seniors.

By incorporating these upper body strength exercises into your routine, you can improve your muscle tone, enhance your posture, and boost your overall strength, allowing you to maintain your independence and perform daily tasks with ease.

Chair Dips

➢ **Why It's Important:**
Chair dips are an effective exercise for strengthening the triceps, which are the muscles located at the back of your upper arms. This exercise helps improve arm strength and contributes to overall upper body stability, making everyday activities like pushing, lifting, and carrying easier.

➢ **How to Perform Chair Dips:**
1. Sit on the edge of a sturdy chair with your feet flat on the floor and your knees bent at a 90-degree angle. Keep your back straight and your shoulders relaxed.
2. Place your hands on the edge of the chair, fingers facing forward, with your palms shoulder-width apart.

3. Inhale deeply and slowly slide your buttocks off the edge of the chair while bending your elbows, lowering your body toward the floor. Keep your elbows close to your body as you lower yourself.
4. Exhale as you push yourself back up to the starting position by straightening your arms. Make sure to engage your core throughout the movement.
5. Repeat the exercise for a total of 8–12 repetitions.

> ## Tips for Chair Dips:

- If you find it difficult to perform the full dip, start with a shallower range of motion by only lowering yourself slightly.
- To increase the challenge, extend your legs further out or place your feet on a second chair.
- Keep your movements controlled to avoid straining your shoulders or elbows.

> ## Benefits:

- Strengthens the triceps, improving arm tone and functionality.
- Enhances upper body stability, making daily tasks easier to perform.
- Promotes better posture by strengthening the muscles that support the shoulders and upper back.

Seated Row

> ## Why It's Important:

The seated row is a fantastic exercise for strengthening the back muscles, particularly the latissimus dorsi, rhomboids, and trapezius. Strengthening these muscles improves posture, reduces back pain, and enhances overall upper body strength, making it easier to perform daily tasks like reaching for objects or carrying groceries.

➢ How to Perform the Seated Row:

1. Sit comfortably in your chair with your back straight and your feet flat on the floor.
2. Use a resistance band or a set of light dumbbells. If using a band, anchor it securely around the legs of the chair or another sturdy object in front of you.
3. Hold the ends of the band or dumbbells with your arms extended in front of you, palms facing each other.
4. Inhale deeply and pull the band or weights toward your torso, bending your elbows and squeezing your shoulder blades together. Keep your elbows close to your sides.
5. Exhale as you slowly return to the starting position, extending your arms forward.
6. Repeat the exercise for a total of 8–12 repetitions.

➢ Tips for Seated Row:

- Maintain a straight back throughout the exercise; avoid leaning forward or arching your back.
- Focus on using your back muscles to pull, rather than relying solely on your arms.
- Adjust the resistance of the band or the weight of the dumbbells to match your strength level.

➢ Benefits:

- Strengthens the back muscles, improving posture and reducing back pain.
- Enhances upper body functionality, making daily activities easier.
- Promotes better core stability and support.

Bicep Curls

> ## Why It's Important:

Bicep curls are a simple yet effective exercise for toning the biceps, the muscles located at the front of your upper arms. Strengthening the biceps contributes to overall arm strength, making it easier to lift and carry objects, as well as improving functional movements in daily life.

> ## How to Perform Bicep Curls:

1. Sit comfortably in your chair with your back straight and your feet flat on the floor. Hold a light dumbbell in each hand, with your arms resting at your sides, palms facing forward.
2. Inhale deeply and slowly lift one dumbbell toward your shoulder, bending your elbow and keeping your upper arm stationary.
3. Exhale as you lower the dumbbell back to the starting position.
4. Repeat the curl with the opposite arm for a total of 8–12 repetitions on each side.
5. If desired, you can perform the exercise simultaneously with both arms.

> ## Tips for Bicep Curls:

- Start with light weights to avoid straining your muscles; you can gradually increase the weight as you become stronger.
- Keep your elbows close to your body throughout the movement; avoid swinging your arms.
- Focus on maintaining a controlled motion, engaging your biceps as you lift the weights.

- ➤ **Benefits:**
- Tones the biceps, improving overall arm strength and appearance.
- Enhances functionality for daily tasks that involve lifting or carrying.
- Promotes better grip strength, which is essential for maintaining independence.

Conclusion

Incorporating upper body strength exercises into your daily routine is essential for maintaining muscle tone, improving posture, and enhancing overall functionality. Chair dips, seated rows, and bicep curls are simple yet effective exercises that require minimal equipment and can be performed in the comfort of your home.

By dedicating just a few minutes each day to these movements, you can significantly improve your upper body strength and overall well-being. Remember, consistency is key; the more you practice these exercises, the greater the benefits you will experience. With a strong upper body, you can enjoy a more active and fulfilling lifestyle, allowing you to participate in daily activities with confidence and ease.

Chapter 07

Lower Body Strength

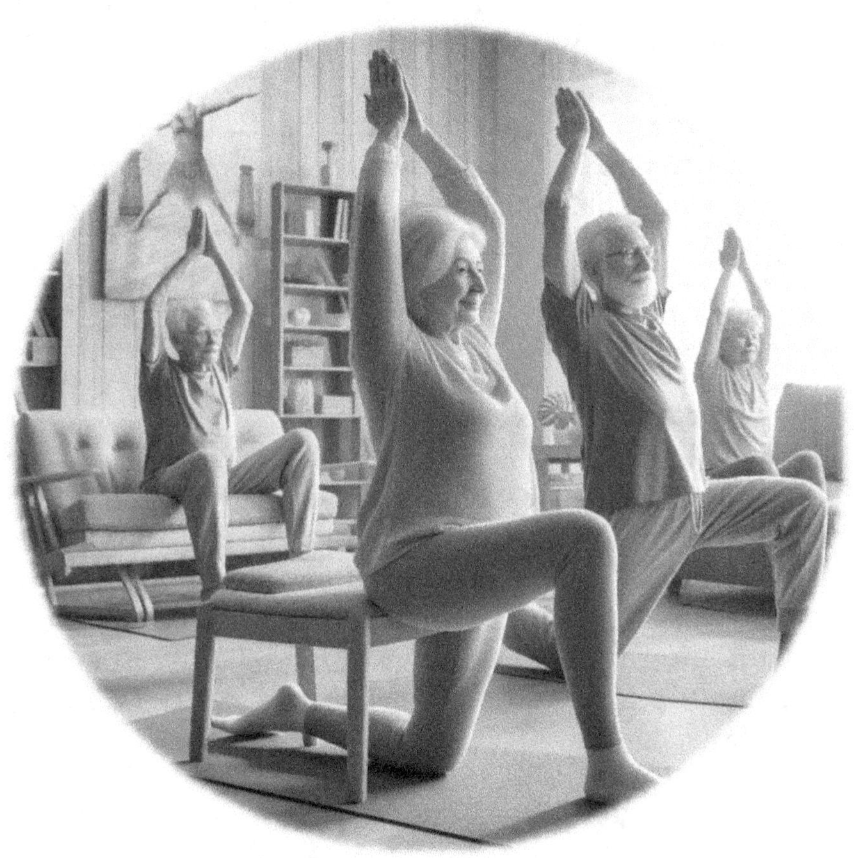

Building and maintaining lower body strength is vital for seniors to enhance mobility, stability, and overall independence. Strong legs and glutes support everyday movements like walking, climbing stairs, and standing up from a seated position. In this chapter, we will explore two effective exercises for strengthening the lower body: chair squats and calf raises. Both exercises are low-impact and can be performed easily from a chair, making them ideal for seniors.

Incorporating these lower body strength exercises into your routine will help improve your functional ability, enhance your balance, and promote a more active lifestyle.

Chair Squats

➢ **Why It's Important:**

Chair squats are an excellent low-impact exercise that targets the quadriceps, hamstrings, and glutes. This functional movement mimics the act of sitting and standing, making it highly relevant to daily life. Strengthening these muscle groups not only enhances leg strength but also improves stability and reduces the risk of falls.

➢ **How to Perform Chair Squats:**
1. Sit at the edge of a sturdy chair with your feet flat on the floor, shoulder-width apart. Keep your back straight and your arms at your sides.
2. Inhale deeply and lean slightly forward, engaging your core muscles.

3. Push through your heels as you rise up from the chair, straightening your legs and keeping your arms extended in front of you for balance.
4. Exhale as you lower yourself back down to the chair, maintaining control as you sit down. Aim to touch the chair lightly with your buttocks without fully sitting down.
5. Repeat the squat for a total of 8–12 repetitions.

➤ Tips for Chair Squats:

- Ensure your chair is stable and won't slide to prevent any accidents.
- Focus on using your legs to lift yourself, avoiding any strain on your back.
- If you find it difficult to lower yourself gently, use your hands to assist in pushing off the chair.

➤ Benefits:

- Strengthens the legs and glutes, improving overall lower body strength.
- Enhances functional movements like standing up, sitting down, and walking.
- Promotes better balance and stability, reducing the risk of falls.

Calf Raises

➤ Why It's Important:

Calf raises are a simple yet effective exercise for targeting the calf muscles (gastrocnemius and soleus). Strong calf muscles play a significant role in walking, running, and maintaining balance. This exercise can enhance lower leg strength and contribute to better overall mobility.

➤ How to Perform Calf Raises:

1. Stand up from your chair, ensuring you have a stable support nearby if needed (such as the back of the chair or a countertop).
2. Place your feet flat on the floor, hip-width apart, with your weight evenly distributed between your feet.
3. Inhale deeply and rise up onto your toes, lifting your heels off the ground. Hold the position at the top for 1–2 seconds.
4. Exhale as you slowly lower your heels back down to the floor.
5. Repeat the calf raise for a total of 10–15 repetitions.

➤ Tips for Calf Raises:

- If you feel comfortable, try performing this exercise without holding onto anything for added challenge.
- Keep your movements slow and controlled to maximize engagement of the calf muscles.
- If you experience discomfort in your ankles or knees, reduce the range of motion or hold onto a support for stability.

➤ Benefits:
- Strengthens the calf muscles, enhancing overall lower leg strength and stability.
- Improves balance and coordination, making walking and standing easier.
- Contributes to better circulation in the lower legs.

Conclusion

Incorporating lower body strength exercises into your daily routine is essential for maintaining muscle tone, improving mobility, and enhancing overall functionality. Chair squats and calf raises are two effective exercises that can be performed easily from the comfort of your home.

By dedicating just a few minutes each day to these movements, you can significantly improve your lower body strength and overall well-being. Remember, consistency is key; the more you practice these exercises, the greater the benefits you will experience. With strong legs and glutes, you can enjoy a more active and fulfilling lifestyle, allowing you to participate in daily activities with confidence and ease.

Part 5:
Cooling Down

Chapter 08

Relaxation Techniques

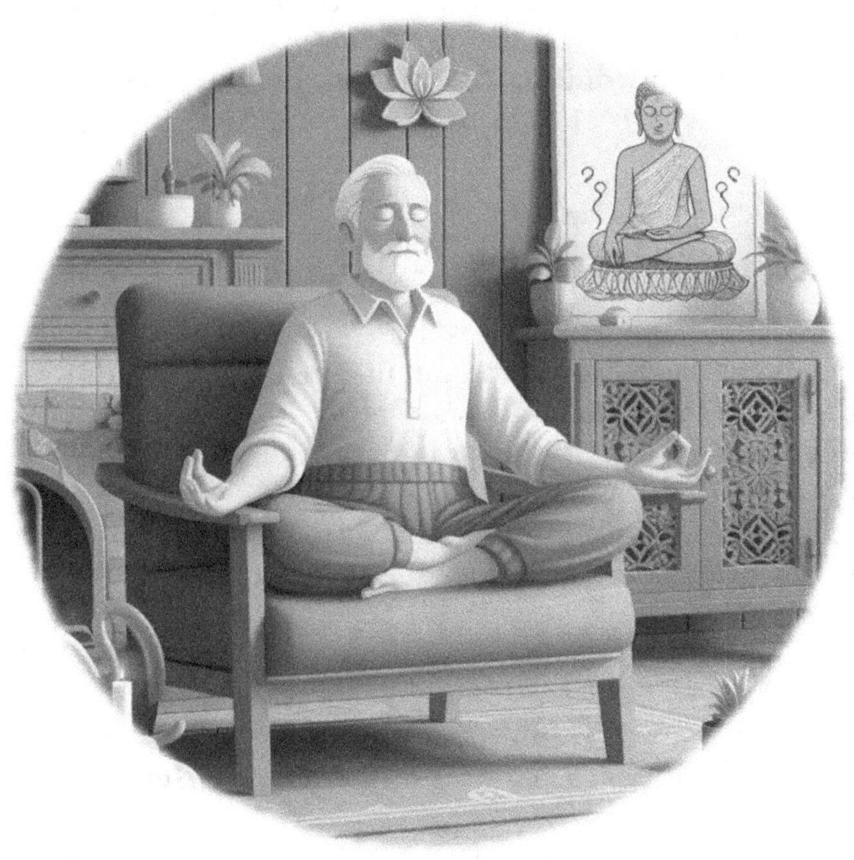

Incorporating relaxation techniques into your daily routine is essential for managing stress, enhancing mental clarity, and promoting overall well-being. For seniors, relaxation techniques can provide numerous benefits, including improved sleep quality, reduced anxiety, and increased feelings of calm. In this chapter, we will explore three effective relaxation techniques: deep breathing, mindfulness meditation, and gentle stretching. Each technique is accessible and can be practiced in a comfortable setting, making them ideal for enhancing relaxation and promoting a sense of peace.

Deep Breathing

➤ Why It's Important:

Deep breathing is a fundamental relaxation technique that activates the body's relaxation response. By engaging in deep, diaphragmatic breathing, you can reduce stress levels, calm your mind, and improve oxygen flow throughout your body. This practice helps lower heart rate and blood pressure, creating a sense of tranquility.

➤ How to Practice Deep Breathing:

1. Find a comfortable position, either sitting in your chair with your feet flat on the floor or lying down if you prefer.
2. Place one hand on your chest and the other on your abdomen. This will help you feel your breath as you inhale and exhale.
3. Inhale deeply through your nose for a count of 4, allowing your abdomen to rise while keeping your chest relatively still.
4. Hold your breath for a count of 4.

5. Exhale slowly through your mouth for a count of 6 or 8, feeling your abdomen fall. Focus on releasing any tension or stress with each exhale.
6. Repeat this process for 5–10 minutes, gradually increasing the duration as you become more comfortable with the technique.

> ## Tips for Deep Breathing:

- Try to practice in a quiet space where you won't be disturbed.
- If you find it difficult to focus, consider counting your breaths or silently repeating a calming word or phrase.
- Practice deep breathing whenever you feel stressed or anxious, or incorporate it into your daily routine to enhance relaxation.

> ## Benefits:
- Reduces stress and anxiety, promoting a sense of calm and well-being.
- Enhances mental clarity and focus by increasing oxygen flow to the brain.
- Improves lung capacity and respiratory function.

Mindfulness Meditation

> ## Why It's Important:
Mindfulness meditation is a powerful technique for promoting relaxation and enhancing mental clarity. By focusing on the present moment without judgment, you can cultivate a sense of peace and calm, reducing feelings of stress and anxiety. Regular mindfulness

practice has been shown to improve emotional well-being and increase overall life satisfaction.

> ## How to Practice Mindfulness Meditation:

1. Find a comfortable position in your chair or a quiet space where you can sit comfortably with your back straight.
2. Close your eyes or keep them softly focused on a spot in front of you.
3. Take a few deep breaths, allowing your body to relax as you inhale and exhale.
4. Bring your attention to the present moment by focusing on your breath. Notice the sensation of the air entering and leaving your body.
5. If your mind begins to wander, gently acknowledge the thoughts without judgment and return your focus to your breath.
6. Continue this practice for 5–15 minutes, gradually increasing the duration as you become more comfortable.

> ## Tips for Mindfulness Meditation:

- Start with shorter sessions (5 minutes) and gradually increase the time as you become more accustomed to the practice.
- Consider using a timer to help you stay focused and avoid distractions.
- If you find it challenging to focus on your breath, you can try a guided meditation or mindfulness app to help you get started.

> ## Benefits:

- Enhances emotional well-being, reducing stress and anxiety.
- Improves focus and concentration, making daily tasks easier to manage.
- Cultivates a sense of self-awareness and mindfulness in everyday life.

Gentle Stretching

> **Why It's Important:**

Gentle stretching is an excellent way to cool down after physical activity and promote relaxation in the body. Stretching helps release tension in the muscles, improves flexibility, and can enhance circulation, contributing to overall well-being. Incorporating gentle stretches into your relaxation routine can help prevent soreness and stiffness, especially after chair yoga sessions.

> **How to Practice Gentle Stretching:**

1. Sit comfortably in your chair with your feet flat on the floor and your back straight.
2. Start with neck stretches:
- Slowly tilt your head to the right, bringing your ear toward your shoulder. Hold for 15–20 seconds and switch sides.
3. Shoulder rolls:
- Roll your shoulders forward in a circular motion for 5–10 repetitions, then reverse the direction.

4. Arm stretches:

- Extend one arm across your body and gently pull it closer with the opposite hand, holding for 15–20 seconds. Switch sides.
5. Seated forward bend:
- While seated, slowly bend forward at your hips, reaching toward the floor or your shins. Hold for 15–30 seconds, breathing deeply as you relax into the stretch.
6. Ankle circles:
- Lift one foot off the ground and rotate your ankle in a circular motion for 5–10 repetitions in each direction. Switch feet.

➤ Tips for Gentle Stretching:

- Focus on your breath during each stretch, inhaling as you prepare to stretch and exhaling as you deepen the stretch.
- Only stretch to the point of mild discomfort; avoid pushing yourself to the point of pain.
- Incorporate gentle stretching into your daily routine, especially after physical activities, to promote relaxation and flexibility.

➤ Benefits:

- Reduces muscle tension, promoting relaxation and reducing stress.
- Enhances flexibility and range of motion, improving overall mobility.
- Supports recovery after physical activity, helping to prevent soreness.

Conclusion

Incorporating relaxation techniques into your daily routine is essential for managing stress, enhancing mental clarity, and promoting overall well-being. Deep breathing, mindfulness meditation, and gentle stretching are effective methods for fostering relaxation and improving your quality of life.

By dedicating just a few minutes each day to these practices, you can cultivate a greater sense of calm and balance in your life. Consistency is key; the more you practice these relaxation techniques, the greater the benefits you will experience. Embrace these techniques as a vital part of your self-care routine, allowing you to navigate life's challenges with greater ease and serenity.

Part 6:
Additional Tips and Considerations

Chapter 09

Nutrition for Seniors

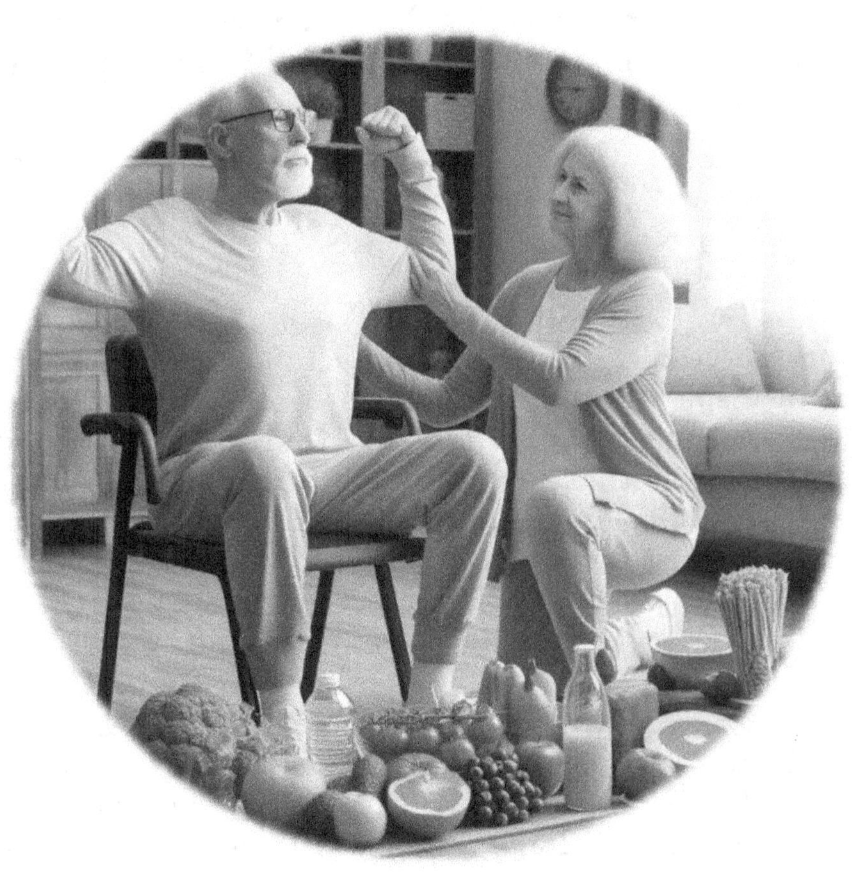

As we age, nutrition becomes increasingly crucial for maintaining health, vitality, and quality of life. A balanced diet provides the essential nutrients our bodies need to function optimally, supports immune health, and helps manage weight. This chapter will explore the importance of a balanced diet for seniors, highlight key nutrients vital for this stage of life, discuss the significance of hydration, and offer tips for practicing mindful eating. By prioritizing nutrition, seniors can enhance their overall well-being and enjoy a healthier, more fulfilling lifestyle.

Balanced Diet

➢ Why It's Important:

A balanced diet is essential for overall health and well-being, especially for seniors. It provides the necessary fuel for energy, supports bodily functions, and helps prevent chronic diseases such as heart disease, diabetes, and osteoporosis. A well-rounded diet should include a variety of food groups, including fruits, vegetables, whole grains, lean proteins, and healthy fats.

➢ Key Components of a Balanced Diet:

1. **Fruits and Vegetables:** Aim to fill half your plate with colorful fruits and vegetables. They are rich in vitamins, minerals, and antioxidants, which can help reduce inflammation and support overall health.

2. **Whole Grains:** Choose whole grains such as brown rice, quinoa, whole wheat bread, and oatmeal. They

provide fiber and essential nutrients, helping to keep your digestive system healthy.

3. **Lean Proteins:** Incorporate sources of lean protein such as chicken, turkey, fish, beans, lentils, and tofu. Protein is essential for maintaining muscle mass and supporting recovery.

4. **Healthy Fats:** Include sources of healthy fats like avocados, nuts, seeds, and olive oil. These fats are beneficial for heart health and can help reduce inflammation.

5. **Dairy or Alternatives:** Ensure you get adequate calcium and vitamin D by including dairy products or fortified alternatives, such as almond or soy milk.

➢ **Tips for Creating a Balanced Plate:**

- Use the "plate method": fill half your plate with fruits and vegetables, one-quarter with lean protein, and one-quarter with whole grains.
- Prepare meals using a variety of colors and textures to enhance visual appeal and ensure a diverse nutrient intake.
- Plan meals ahead of time to avoid last-minute unhealthy choices.

Essential Nutrients

➢ **Why They Matter:**

As we age, our nutritional needs change. Certain nutrients become more critical for maintaining health and preventing age-related conditions. Here are some essential nutrients that seniors should prioritize:

1. Calcium:

- Importance: Essential for maintaining bone health and preventing osteoporosis.
- Sources: Dairy products, leafy greens (like kale and broccoli), fortified plant-based milks, and tofu.

2. Vitamin D:

- Importance: Supports calcium absorption and promotes bone health. It also plays a role in immune function.
- Sources: Fatty fish (salmon, mackerel), fortified foods (like cereals and orange juice), and sunlight exposure.

3. Protein:

- Importance: Necessary for maintaining muscle mass, repairing tissues, and supporting immune function.
- Sources: Lean meats, poultry, fish, eggs, legumes, nuts, and dairy.

4. Fiber:

- Importance: Aids in digestion, helps maintain healthy cholesterol levels, and can prevent constipation.
- Sources: Whole grains, fruits, vegetables, legumes, and nuts.

➤ **Practical Ways to Increase Essential Nutrients:**

- Add a serving of leafy greens to your meals (e.g., salads, smoothies).

- Incorporate a variety of protein sources throughout the week, including plant-based options.
- Choose whole grain products over refined grains to increase fiber intake.

Hydration

> ## Why It's Important:

Staying hydrated is essential for seniors, as the body's ability to sense thirst diminishes with age. Adequate hydration supports digestion, nutrient absorption, temperature regulation, and overall bodily functions. Dehydration can lead to serious health issues, including kidney problems, urinary tract infections, and confusion.

> ## Tips for Staying Hydrated:

1. Drink Water Regularly: Aim for at least 8 cups of water a day. Carry a water bottle with you to encourage frequent sipping.
2. Include Hydrating Foods: Foods like cucumbers, watermelon, oranges, and soups can contribute to your daily fluid intake.
3. Set Reminders: Use alarms or phone apps to remind you to drink water throughout the day.
4. Limit Caffeinated and Alcoholic Beverages: Both can contribute to dehydration, so balance them with plenty of water.

> ## Signs of Dehydration:
- Dry mouth or throat
- Dark yellow urine

- Fatigue or dizziness
- Confusion or irritability

Mindful Eating

> **Why It's Important:**

Mindful eating is a practice that encourages awareness of your eating habits and the sensory experience of eating. This technique can help prevent overeating, improve digestion, and enhance enjoyment of meals. By being present during meals, seniors can make healthier choices and develop a better relationship with food.

> **Tips for Practicing Mindful Eating:**

1. **Slow Down:** Take your time to chew your food thoroughly and savor each bite. Aim to put your utensils down between bites to encourage slower eating.

2. **Eliminate Distractions:** Turn off the TV and put away your phone during meals. Focus on your food and the experience of eating.

3. **Listen to Your Body:** Pay attention to hunger and fullness cues. Eat when you're hungry, and stop when you're satisfied, even if there's food left on your plate.

4. **Appreciate Your Food:** Take a moment to acknowledge where your food comes from. Consider the colors, textures, and flavors of what you're eating.

5. Practice Gratitude: Before starting a meal, express gratitude for the food and the effort it took to prepare it. This practice can enhance your enjoyment of meals.

- Promotes healthier food choices by encouraging awareness of what you're consuming.
- Reduces emotional eating, helping you develop a healthier relationship with food.
- Enhances digestion by promoting slower eating and mindful chewing.

Conclusion

Nutrition plays a vital role in maintaining health and well-being for seniors. A balanced diet rich in essential nutrients, combined with proper hydration and mindful eating practices, can significantly enhance quality of life. By prioritizing these nutritional strategies, seniors can support their physical health, improve energy levels, and reduce the risk of chronic diseases.

Embrace these nutrition principles as part of your daily routine, and take the time to explore new recipes and food options that nourish your body and delight your taste buds. Remember, small changes can lead to significant improvements in your overall health and vitality. By investing in your nutrition, you are investing in a healthier, happier future.

Chapter 10

Incorporating Chair Yoga into Daily Life

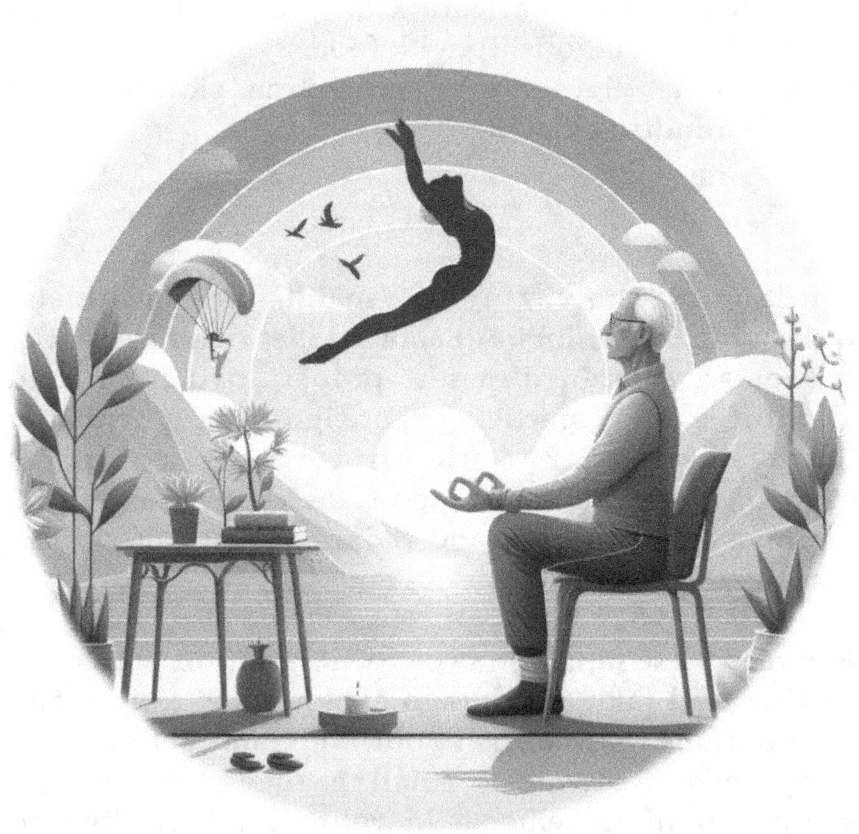

Integrating chair yoga into your daily routine can transform your health and well-being, especially as you navigate the challenges of aging. Regular practice can enhance your flexibility, strength, and mental clarity, and help you maintain a positive outlook on life. This chapter will provide actionable strategies for establishing a consistent chair yoga routine, the benefits of finding a practice partner, tips for overcoming common challenges, and the importance of celebrating your progress along the way.

Creating a Routine

➢ Establishing a Consistent Practice

Creating a routine is key to reaping the benefits of chair yoga. Here are some effective strategies to help you incorporate chair yoga into your daily life:

1. Set Specific Goals:

- Decide what you want to achieve through chair yoga. Whether it's improved flexibility, reduced stress, or enhanced strength, having clear goals will keep you motivated.
- Write down your goals and place them somewhere visible as a reminder.

2. Choose a Regular Time:

- Determine a specific time each day that works best for you, whether it's in the morning, afternoon, or evening.
- Treat this time as an important appointment for your health. Consistency helps develop a habit.

3. Create a Dedicated Space:

- Designate a comfortable, quiet space in your home for your chair yoga practice. This could be a corner of your living room or a sunlit area.
- Keep your chair, yoga props, and any additional items organized and easily accessible.

4. Start Small:

- If you're new to chair yoga, begin with short sessions — 10 to 15 minutes a day. Gradually increase the duration as you become more comfortable.
- Consistency is more important than length; it's better to practice regularly for shorter periods than to do long sessions infrequently.

5. Use a Calendar or Journal:

- Keep a calendar or journal to track your chair yoga sessions. Note the date, duration, and how you felt afterward.
- This can help you stay accountable and also allows you to reflect on your progress over time.

➢ Creating a Structured Session

When establishing your routine, consider the following structure for your chair yoga practice:

- Warm-Up (2-3 minutes): Start with gentle neck and shoulder stretches to prepare your body.
- Main Practice (5-10 minutes): Focus on specific poses and stretches that target your goals (e.g., balance, flexibility).
- Cool Down (2-3 minutes): Conclude with relaxation techniques, such as deep breathing or gentle stretching.

By following a structured session, you will build familiarity and make your practice feel more intentional.

Finding a Practice Partner

> ➤ **The Benefits of Practicing with a Partner or Group:**

Practicing chair yoga with a partner or in a group setting can enhance your experience in several ways:

1. Accountability:
- Having a partner helps you stay committed to your practice. When you know someone else is counting on you, you're more likely to show up.
- Schedule regular sessions together, whether it's once a week or a few times a week.

2. Social Interaction:
- Practicing with others can foster social connections and reduce feelings of isolation, which can be common in later life.
- Sharing experiences and progress can create a sense of community and support.

3. Motivation and Encouragement:
- A partner can provide encouragement when you're feeling unmotivated, helping you push through barriers.
- You can inspire each other to explore new poses or techniques, making the practice more enjoyable.

4. Learning Opportunities:

- Practicing together allows you to learn from each other. You may discover new techniques or modifications that can enhance your practice.
- Consider joining a local chair yoga class or community center where you can meet others with similar interests.

➢ **Finding a Suitable Partner**

- Family and Friends: Invite family members or friends to join you in your practice. This can be a fun bonding experience.
- Community Groups: Check local community centers, senior centers, or fitness studios for chair yoga classes or groups.
- Online Platforms: Explore virtual classes where you can practice with others from the comfort of your home.

Overcoming Challenges

➢ **Common Barriers to Regular Practice**

While chair yoga offers many benefits, it's not uncommon to face challenges along the way. Here are tips for overcoming some of the most common obstacles:

1. Lack of Motivation:

- Set Reminders: Use phone alerts or sticky notes to remind you of your scheduled practice time.

- Variety in Routine: Keep your practice fresh by varying the poses and techniques you use. Explore different online classes or apps for inspiration.
- Visualize Benefits: Focus on how good you feel after practicing. Keeping that feeling in mind can help reignite your motivation.

2. Physical Limitations:

- Listen to Your Body: It's essential to listen to your body and respect its limits. If a pose feels uncomfortable, modify it or skip it.
- Seek Guidance: If you have concerns about your abilities, consider consulting with a healthcare provider or certified yoga instructor who can provide tailored advice and modifications.
- Focus on What You Can Do: Shift your mindset to what you can achieve rather than what you can't. Celebrate your unique abilities.

3. Time Constraints:

- Short Sessions: If you're busy, focus on shorter practices that fit your schedule. Even a 5-minute session can be beneficial.
- Integrate into Daily Activities: Incorporate chair yoga into other daily activities, such as during TV time or while reading.

4. Boredom:

- Mix It Up: Change your routine or try new poses to keep things interesting. Experiment with different times of day for practice to find what feels best.

- Join Classes: Participating in live classes can bring excitement and structure to your practice.

Celebrating Progress

➢ Acknowledging Your Achievements

Recognizing and celebrating your progress is crucial for maintaining motivation and reinforcing positive behaviors. Here's how you can celebrate your achievements effectively:

1. Set Milestones:

- Break your larger goals into smaller, achievable milestones. For instance, aim to practice consistently for a week or master a new pose.
- Celebrate each milestone with a small reward, such as treating yourself to a favorite healthy snack or taking a day off to relax.

2. Track Your Progress:

- Keep a journal or log to document your practice sessions, how you felt, and any improvements you've noticed over time.
- Regularly review your entries to see how far you've come, which can serve as motivation to continue.

3. Share Your Journey:

- Share your experiences with friends, family, or a community group. Talking about your journey can inspire others and foster a supportive environment.

- Consider creating a social media group where you can post updates and connect with fellow chair yoga enthusiasts.

4. Reflect on Your Benefits:

- Take time to reflect on the benefits you've experienced since starting chair yoga. This could include improved flexibility, reduced stress, or enhanced balance.
- Keep a gratitude journal to note specific ways chair yoga has positively impacted your life, reinforcing the value of your practice.

5. Embrace Each Session:

- Recognize that every session, no matter how short or challenging, contributes to your overall well-being.
- Celebrate simply by acknowledging the time you dedicated to your health, regardless of the outcomes.

Conclusion

Incorporating chair yoga into your daily life can significantly enhance your physical and mental well-being. By establishing a consistent routine, finding a practice partner, overcoming challenges, and celebrating your progress, you can create a fulfilling chair yoga practice that supports your journey to feeling younger, stronger, and healthier.

Embrace the practice as a powerful tool to enrich your life, and remember that every small step counts. With determination and positivity, you can make chair yoga an integral part of your daily routine, leading to improved health and a greater sense of vitality.

Conclusion

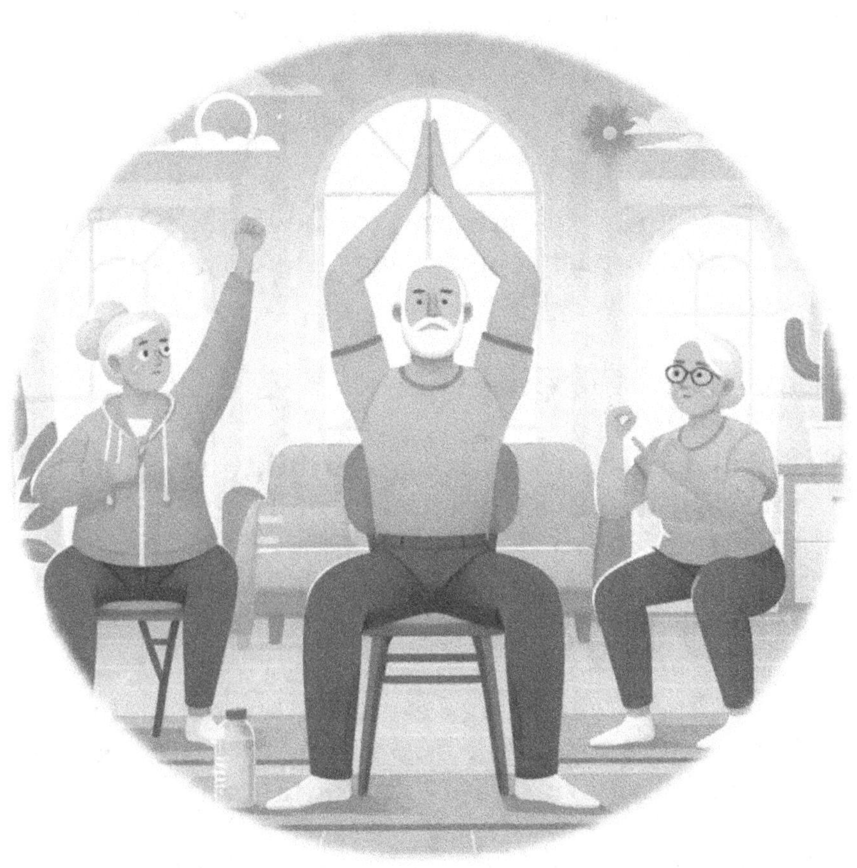

As we conclude this journey through the transformative world of chair yoga, let's take a moment to reflect on the numerous benefits it offers, especially for seniors. The accessibility and adaptability of chair yoga make it a perfect choice for anyone seeking to enhance their physical health, mental well-being, and overall quality of life.

Recap of Benefits

Chair yoga provides an array of advantages that can significantly impact seniors' lives. Here's a recap of the key benefits:

1.Improved Flexibility:

- Regular practice enhances flexibility in joints and muscles, helping to maintain mobility and reduce the risk of injury.

2. Increased Strength:

- Engaging in chair yoga exercises builds strength in key muscle groups, contributing to better balance and stability, which are vital for fall prevention.

3. Enhanced Balance and Coordination:

- Through specific poses and movements, chair yoga improves overall body awareness, leading to better balance and coordination.

4. Pain Relief and Reduced Stiffness:

- Gentle stretches and movements alleviate tension and stiffness in the body, making daily activities more comfortable.

5. Stress Reduction and Mental Clarity:

- Incorporating mindfulness and relaxation techniques in chair yoga promotes mental clarity, reduces stress, and enhances emotional well-being.

6. Social Interaction:

- Practicing chair yoga in groups fosters social connections and community support, which can combat feelings of isolation.

7. Convenience and Accessibility:

- Chair yoga can be done at home, in a group setting, or virtually, making it accessible for those with limited mobility or space.

8. Better Posture:

- Regular practice helps to strengthen core muscles and improve posture, reducing strain on the back and neck.

9. Enhanced Quality of Life:

- The combination of physical, mental, and social benefits contributes to an improved overall quality of life, allowing seniors to engage more fully in activities they love.

Encouragement to Continue

As you conclude this guide, remember that the journey toward better health and well-being through chair yoga is ongoing. The benefits mentioned above are not just short-term gains but are enhanced by consistent practice. Here are some motivational reminders to keep you on track:

- **Start Small, Dream Big:** Each time you engage in chair yoga, no matter how brief, you are taking a significant step towards your health goals. Focus on the process rather than perfection, and celebrate each session as a victory.

- **Be Patient with Yourself:** Progress may be gradual, but every small improvement counts. Trust the journey and remain patient with your body as it adapts and evolves.

- **Stay Curious:** Explore new poses, techniques, and resources. Keep your practice fresh and exciting by trying different styles of chair yoga or joining classes with varied approaches.

- **Listen to Your Body:** Respect your limits and make modifications as needed. Your body is your best guide, and honoring it will lead to a more fulfilling practice.

- **Remember Your Why:** Revisit the reasons you started chair yoga. Whether it's to improve health, connect with others, or enhance quality of life, keeping your motivation in mind will help sustain your practice.

Resources and Recommendations

To further support your chair yoga journey, consider the following resources and recommendations:

1. Online Classes and Videos:

- Websites like YouTube and dedicated yoga platforms offer a range of chair yoga classes suitable for different levels. Search for reputable instructors who specialize in chair yoga for seniors.

2. Books and Guides:

- Explore literature focused on chair yoga, which often includes illustrations and detailed instructions for poses. Titles like "Chair Yoga: Sitting Poses for Everyone" can provide additional insights and inspiration.

3. Local Community Centers:

- Check local community centers, senior centers, or fitness studios for chair yoga classes. Practicing in a group setting can enhance motivation and provide a sense of community.

4. Yoga Apps:

- Download yoga apps that offer chair yoga programs. Many apps include features like guided sessions, progress tracking, and community forums to connect with other practitioners.

5. Social Media Groups:

- Join online communities or social media groups dedicated to chair yoga. These platforms offer support, motivation, and opportunities to share your journey with others.

6. Consult a Professional:

- If you have specific health concerns or conditions, consider consulting a healthcare provider or certified yoga instructor who specializes in chair yoga for personalized guidance.

7. Mindfulness and Meditation Resources:

- Explore resources that focus on mindfulness and meditation techniques. Integrating these practices can enhance the mental benefits of chair yoga.

8. Create Your Own Routine:

- Use the knowledge gained from this guide to develop a personalized chair yoga routine that fits your needs and lifestyle. Experiment with different sequences and durations to find what works best for you.

As you embrace chair yoga, remember that it's more than just a form of exercise; it's a pathway to a healthier, happier life. By integrating chair yoga into your daily routine, you're investing in your long-term health and well-being. Continue to explore, practice, and celebrate every step of your journey toward feeling younger, stronger, and healthier. Your commitment to chair yoga is a powerful gift to yourself—embrace it fully!

www.ingramcontent.com/pod-product-compliance
Lightning Source LLC
Chambersburg PA
CBHW050819250726
48653CB00006B/2312